The Easy Gastroparesis Cookbook

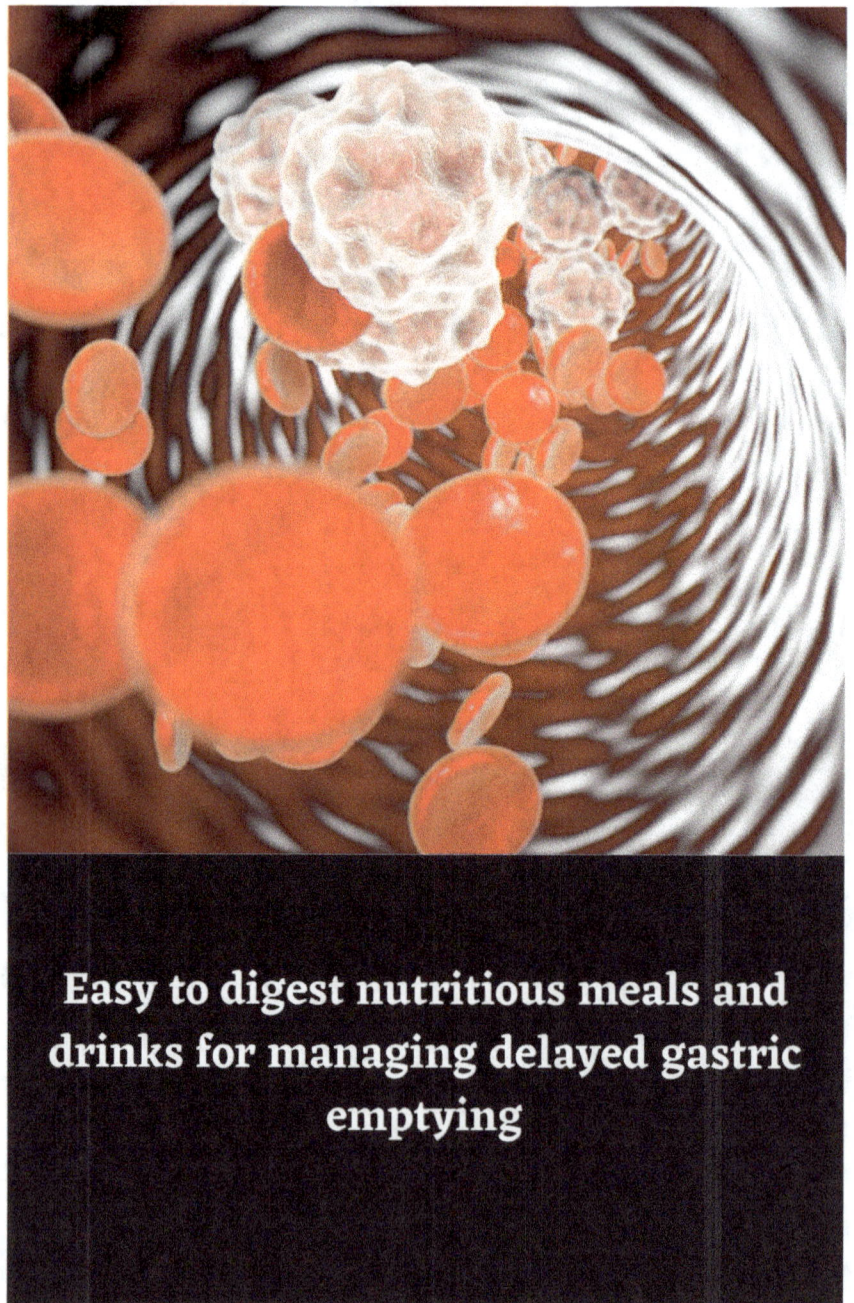

Easy to digest nutritious meals and drinks for managing delayed gastric emptying

DEDICATION

This book is dedicated to everyone battling gastroparesis and looking for solutions to enhance their diets while still indulging in sumptuous meals and drinks.

ACKNOWLEDGMENTS

We would like to thank the gastroparesis community for their invaluable suggestions, comments, and assistance throughout the writing of this book. We also want to express our gratitude to the doctors and nurses who put forth so much effort to make the lives of people with gastroparesis better. Finally, we want to express our gratitude to our family and friends for their constant support and faith in our mission.

TABLE OF CONTENT

Introduction

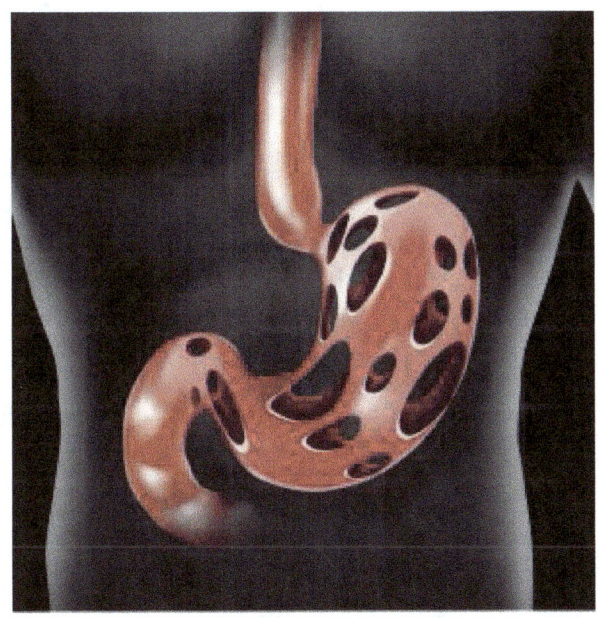

What is gastroparesis?

When you have gastroparesis, your stomach's normal rate of emptying into your small intestine is slowed down. The reason for this is because your stomach muscles aren't functioning correctly. It may be an unpleasant and difficult illness to live with, but there are solutions available to help control the symptoms.

Symptoms of gastroparesis

The most well-known sign of gastroparesis is likely nausea. You could feel like throwing up because of the nauseous sensation in your stomach. Sadly, nausea often causes vomiting in patients with gastroparesis. Undigested food from hours or even days earlier may come up in your vomit because the stomach is not emptying correctly. Ugh, I know.

- Bloating in the abdomen: Your stomach may begin to feel like a balloon that is ready to burst when it cannot empty correctly. Your stomach may feel uncomfortable or even hurt as a result.
- Speaking of discomfort, some gastroparesis sufferers may feel a severe or mild ache in their belly. Gas accumulation and other stomach contents may be to blame for this.
- Feeling full after just a few bites: Feeling full after only a few bites of food is another typical symptom of gastroparesis. It might be irritating and challenging to get the nutrients you need because of this.
- Acid reflux: When your stomach is unable to empty completely, it may result in acid reflux (commonly referred to as heartburn) because the stomach acid backs up into the esophagus.
- Changes in blood sugar levels: If you have diabetes, gastroparesis may also have an impact on your blood sugar levels. Managing your blood sugar may be more challenging since your stomach is not emptying completely.

Causes of gastroparesis

One of the most prevalent causes of gastroparesis is diabetes. The nerves that regulate the muscles in your stomach may be harmed by high blood sugar levels, making it more difficult for your stomach to empty completely.

- Surgery: Gastroparesis may sometimes result after stomach or intestinal surgery. This is due to the possibility that the procedure would harm the nerves that regulate your stomach's muscles

- Medication: A gastroparesis-causing medicine might slow down the passage of food through your stomach and intestines. Opioids, antidepressants, and several medicines used to treat high blood pressure are some of the most popular drugs that might cause this.
- Neurological conditions: Conditions like Parkinson's disease or multiple sclerosis may potentially contribute to gastroparesis. The nerves that regulate the muscles in your stomach may be harmed by these disorders. In rare instances, a viral illness like the flu or herpes may lead to gastroparesis. The nerves that control the muscles in your stomach may get damaged due to the illness.
- Gastroparesis may also occur in people who have eating disorders like anorexia or bulimia. This is due to the fact that bingeing and purging repeatedly might harm your stomach's muscles.

Diagnosis and treatment options

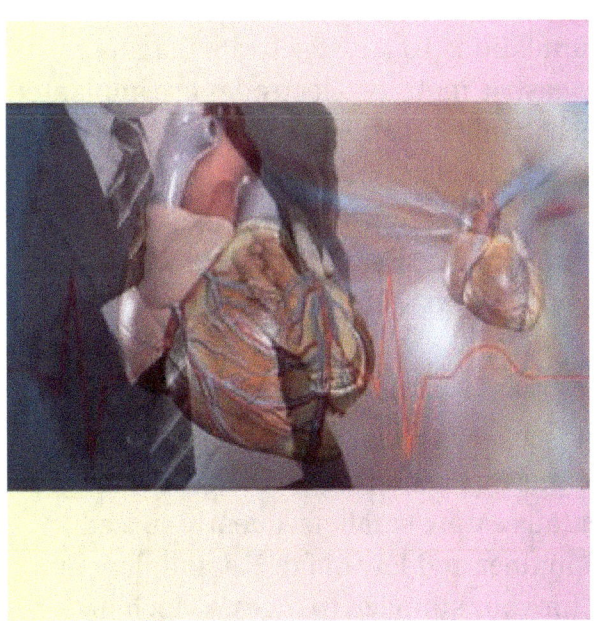

- Gastric emptying study: This is a test that examines how fast food exits your stomach and enters your small intestine. It entails consuming a meal that contains a tiny quantity of radioactive material, followed by scans that are performed at spaced-apart periods to monitor the movement of the food.

- Upper endoscopy: This is a technique in which a flexible tube with a camera on the end is placed into your mouth and down your neck to check your esophagus, stomach, and upper small intestine.
- Blood testing: In order to rule out underlying diseases that may be causing your symptoms, your doctor may prescribe blood tests.

There are several treatment options available when a gastroparesis diagnosis has been made, including:

- Changing your diet to include smaller, more often meals and stay away from high-fiber and high-fat foods will assist with gastroparesis symptoms.
- Metoclopramide and erythromycin are a few of the drugs that may help make it easier for food to go through your stomach.
- Electrical stimulation: To assist activate the muscles and enhance gastric motility, electrodes are implanted in the stomach's wall and attached to a machine that transmits electrical pulses.
- Surgery: In very rare circumstances, surgery may be required to remove scar tissue or repair damage to the nerves that control your stomach muscles.

What is a diet for gastroparesis?

A gastroparesis diet is an eating plan that may help you manage your symptoms by facilitating food digestion in your stomach. It often entails eating small, frequently spaced meals that are high in fiber and low in fat. Fat and fiber are both more difficult for your stomach to digest, which may make sensations like bloating and nausea worse. Instead, the emphasis should be on consuming simple-to-digest meals like lean protein, steamed veggies, and low-fat dairy.

What food is best?

It's crucial to choose meals that are simple to digest while on a gastroparesis diet. Here are several examples:

- Eggs, chicken, fish, turkey, tofu, and other lean proteins
- cooked vegetables: potatoes, squash, green beans, and carrots
- Low-fat dairy products include milk, yogurt, and cheese.
- White rice, white bread, and pasta are grains.
- Fruits: fresh, cooked, or canned (avoid raw fruits)
- Little quantities of olive oil or butter for fats

Eating small frequent meals throughout the day is preferable than a few big ones. This may prevent your stomach from being overstuffed, which can make your symptoms worse.

What should you stay away from?

Certain foods should be avoided on a gastroparesis diet because they are more difficult for your stomach to absorb. Here are several examples:

- Meals high in fat: fried items, fatty meats, and creamy sauces
- Foods high in fiber: whole grains, uncooked veggies, beans, and lentils
- Drinks with carbonation: soda and sparkling water
- Beer, wine, and spirits
- Avoid consuming a lot of food at once by avoiding

large meals.

Also, it's crucial to refrain from eating too rapidly and from laying down shortly after eating. These two factors have the potential to worsen symptoms.

Tips for meal planning

When you follow a gastroparesis diet, meal planning might be a bit challenging, but there are several strategies that can help:

- Prepare your meals in advance to ensure that you obtain a decent mix of nutrients and stay away from items that make your symptoms worse.
- Consume meals slowly and thoroughly to facilitate easy digestion in your stomach.
- Consume beverages separately from meals to avoid overfilling your stomach.
- Maintain a meal journal to help you identify the foods that make you feel sick so you can avoid them in the future.

Chapter 1: Breakfast Ideas

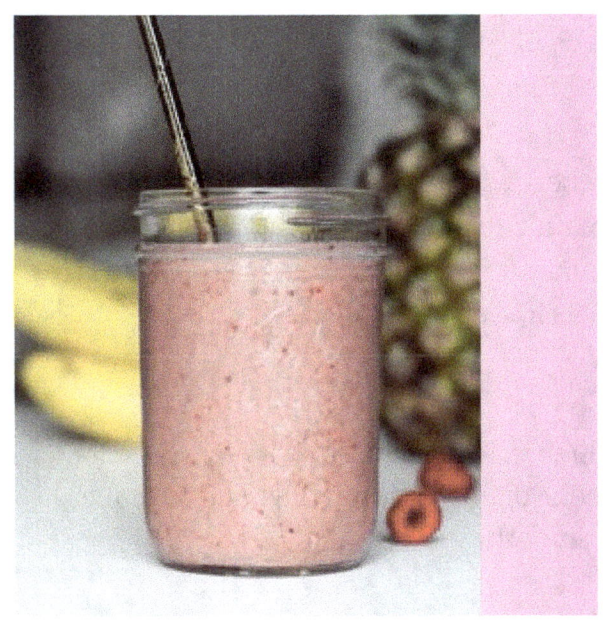

SMOOTHIES AND SHAKES

Banana and Peanut Butter Smoothie

Ingredients:

- 1 ripe banana
- 1 tablespoon of peanut butter
- 1/2 cup of almond milk
- 1/2 cup of ice cubes

Cooking Guidelines :

1) Cut the banana into small pieces and place it in a blender.
2) Add the peanut butter, almond milk, and ice cubes.
3) Blend until smooth.
4) Serve.

Blueberry and Yogurt Smoothie

Ingredients:

- 1 cup of blueberries
- 1/2 cup of plain Greek yogurt
- 1/2 cup of almond milk
- 1/2 cup of ice cubes

Cooking Guidelines :

1) Rinse the blueberries and place them in a blender.
2) Add the Greek yogurt, almond milk, and ice cubes.
3) Blend until smooth.
4) Serve.

Banana and Oatmeal Shake

Ingredients:

- 1 ripe banana

- 1/2 cup of cooked oatmeal
- 1/2 cup of almond milk
- 1/2 teaspoon of vanilla extract
- 1/2 cup of ice cubes

Cooking Guidelines :

1) Cut the banana into small pieces and place it in a blender.
2) Add the cooked oatmeal, almond milk, vanilla extract, and ice cubes.
3) Blend until smooth.
4) Serve.

Pumpkin Pie Smoothie

Ingredients:

- 1/2 cup of canned pumpkin puree
- 1/2 cup of plain Greek yogurt
- 1/2 cup of almond milk
- 1/2 teaspoon of pumpkin pie spice
- 1/2 cup of ice cubes

Cooking Guidelines :

1) In a blender, combine the pumpkin puree, Greek yogurt, almond milk, pumpkin pie spice, and ice cubes.
2) Blend until smooth.
3) Serve.

Strawberry and Banana Smoothie

Ingredients:

- 1 ripe banana
- 1 cup of frozen strawberries
- 1/2 cup of plain Greek yogurt
- 1/2 cup of almond milk
- 1/2 cup of ice cubes

Cooking Guidelines :

1) Cut the banana into small pieces and place it in a blender.
2) Add the frozen strawberries, Greek yogurt, almond milk, and ice cubes
3) Blend until smooth
4) Serve.

OATMEAL AND PORRIDGE

Cinnamon and Apple Oatmeal

Ingredients:

- 1/2 cup of rolled oats
- 1 cup of water
- 1/2 teaspoon of cinnamon
- 1/2 apple, diced
- 1 tablespoon of honey

Cooking Guidelines :

1) In a saucepan, combine the rolled oats, water, and cinnamon.
2) Bring to a boil over medium heat.

3) Reduce the heat to low and add the diced apple.
4) Cook for 5-7 minutes, stirring occasionally.
5) Remove from heat and stir in the honey.
6) Serve warm.

Blueberry and Almond Porridge

Ingredients:

- 1/2 cup of rolled oats
- 1 cup of almond milk
- 1/2 cup of blueberries
- 1 tablespoon of almond butter
- 1 teaspoon of honey

Cooking Guidelines :

1) In a saucepan, combine the rolled oats and almond milk.
2) Bring to a boil over medium heat.
3) Reduce the heat to low and add the blueberries.
4) Cook for 5-7 minutes, stirring occasionally.
5) Remove from heat and stir in the almond butter and honey.
6) Serve warm.

Banana and Peanut Butter Oatmeal

Ingredients:

- 1/2 cup of rolled oats
- 1 cup of water
- 1/2 banana, sliced

- 1 tablespoon of peanut butter
- 1 teaspoon of honey

Cooking Guidelines :

1) In a saucepan, combine the rolled oats and water.
2) Bring to a boil over medium heat.
3) Reduce the heat to low and add the sliced banana.
4) Cook for 5-7 minutes, stirring occasionally.
5) Remove from heat and stir in the peanut butter and honey.
6) Serve warm.

Pumpkin Spice Porridge

Ingredients:

- 1/2 cup of rolled oats
- 1 cup of almond milk
- 1/4 cup of pumpkin puree
- 1/2 teaspoon of pumpkin pie spice
- 1 tablespoon of maple syrup

Cooking Guidelines :

1) In a saucepan, combine the rolled oats and almond milk.
2) Bring to a boil over medium heat.
3) Reduce the heat to low and add the pumpkin puree and pumpkin pie spice.
4) Cook for 5-7 minutes, stirring occasionally.
5) Remove from heat and stir in the maple syrup.
6) Serve warm.

Peach and Vanilla Oatmeal

Ingredients:

- 1/2 cup of rolled oats
- 1 cup of water
- 1/2 peach, sliced
- 1/2 teaspoon of vanilla extract
- 1 teaspoon of honey

Cooking Guidelines :

1) In a saucepan, combine the rolled oats and water.
2) Bring to a boil over medium heat.
3) Reduce the heat to low and add the sliced peach and vanilla extract.
4) Cook for 5-7 minutes, stirring occasionally.
5) Remove from heat and stir in the honey.
6) Serve warm.

EGG-BASED DISHES

Soft-Boiled Eggs with Toast

Ingredients:

- 2 eggs
- 2 slices of whole-grain toast
- Salt and pepper to taste

Cooking Guidelines :

1) Bring a small pot of water to a boil.

2) Gently place the eggs in the boiling water and cook for 6 minutes.
3) Remove the eggs from the pot and rinse them under cold water to stop the cooking process.
4) Serve the eggs with the toast, and sprinkle with salt and pepper.

Scrambled Eggs with Spinach and Feta

Ingredients:

- 2 eggs
- 1/4 cup of fresh spinach, chopped
- 1 tablespoon of crumbled feta cheese
- Salt and pepper to taste

Cooking Guidelines :

1) Crack the eggs into a bowl and whisk them together.
2) In a non-stick pan, sauté the spinach until wilted.
3) Pour the eggs into the pan and stir gently with a spatula.
4) Cook until the eggs are set, but still moist.
5) Sprinkle with feta cheese and season with salt and pepper.

Veggie Omelet

Ingredients:

- 2 eggs
- 1/4 cup of diced red bell pepper
- 1/4 cup of diced zucchini

- 1 tablespoon of olive oil
- Salt and pepper to taste

Cooking Guidelines :

1) Crack the eggs into a bowl and whisk them together.
2) In a non-stick pan, heat the olive oil over medium-high heat.
3) Sauté the red bell pepper and zucchini until they are softened.
4) Pour the eggs into the pan and let cook for a minute or two.
5) When the edges of the eggs begin to set, use a spatula to fold the omelet in half.
6) Cook for an additional minute or two, until the eggs are set.
7) Season with salt and pepper.

Baked Eggs with Tomatoes and Basil

Ingredients:

- 2 eggs
- 1/2 cup of diced tomatoes
- 1 tablespoon of chopped fresh basil
- Salt and pepper to taste

Cooking Guidelines :

1) Preheat the oven to 375°F (190°C).
2) Crack the eggs into a small oven-safe dish.
3) Add the diced tomatoes and chopped basil to the dish.
4) Bake for 10-15 minutes, or until the eggs are set.
5) Season with salt and pepper.

Egg Drop Soup

Ingredients:

- 2 cups of chicken or vegetable broth
- 2 eggs, beaten
- 1 green onion, thinly sliced
- Salt and pepper to taste

Cooking Guidelines :

1) In a pot, bring the broth to a simmer.
2) Slowly pour the beaten eggs into the broth, while stirring constantly with a fork.
3) Cook for 1-2 minutes, until the eggs are set.
4) Add the sliced green onion and season with salt and pepper.
5) Serve hot.

GLUTEN-FREE AND DAIRY-FREE OPTIONS

Quinoa and Roasted Vegetable Salad

Ingredients:

- 1 cup of cooked quinoa
- 1 cup of roasted vegetables (such as zucchini, bell peppers, and sweet potatoes)
- 2 tablespoons of chopped fresh herbs (such as parsley or cilantro)
- 1 tablespoon of olive oil
- 1 tablespoon of balsamic vinegar

- Salt and pepper to taste

Cooking Guidelines :

1) In a bowl, mix together the cooked quinoa, roasted vegetables, and chopped herbs.
2) In a separate bowl, whisk together the olive oil and balsamic vinegar to make the dressing.
3) Pour the dressing over the quinoa and vegetables and toss to coat.
4) Season with salt and pepper to taste.

Grilled Chicken and Vegetable Skewers

Ingredients:

- 1 chicken breast, cut into bite-sized pieces
- 1 cup of vegetables (such as cherry tomatoes, zucchini, and bell peppers)
- 1 tablespoon of olive oil
- Salt and pepper to taste

Cooking Guidelines :

1) Preheat a grill or grill pan to medium-high heat.
2) Thread the chicken and vegetables onto skewers.
3) Brush the skewers with olive oil and season with salt and pepper.
4) Grill the skewers for 8-10 minutes, or until the chicken is cooked through and the vegetables are tender.

Baked Salmon with Roasted Vegetables

Ingredients:

- 1 salmon fillet
- 1 cup of roasted vegetables (such as asparagus, broccoli, and carrots)
- 1 tablespoon of olive oil
- Salt and pepper to taste

Cooking Guidelines :

1) Preheat the oven to 375°F (190°C).
2) Place the salmon fillet in a baking dish.
3) Toss the roasted vegetables with olive oil and season with salt and pepper.
4) Arrange the vegetables around the salmon in the baking dish.
5) Bake for 15-20 minutes, or until the salmon is cooked through and the vegetables are tender.

Green Smoothie Bowl

Ingredients:

- 1 banana, sliced
- 1 cup of spinach
- 1/2 cup of frozen mango chunks
- 1/2 cup of unsweetened almond milk
- Toppings (such as sliced strawberries, chia seeds, and shredded coconut)

Cooking Guidelines :

1) In a blender, combine the banana, spinach, mango chunks, and almond milk.
2) Blend until smooth.

3) Pour the smoothie into a bowl.
4) Top with sliced strawberries, chia seeds, and shredded coconut.

Vegetable Stir-Fry with Rice

Ingredients:

- 1 cup of cooked brown rice
- 1 cup of mixed vegetables (such as bell peppers, broccoli, and carrots)
- 1 tablespoon of coconut oil
- 1 tablespoon of gluten-free tamari sauce
- Salt and pepper to taste

Cooking Guidelines :

1) In a large skillet or wok, heat the coconut oil over high heat.
2) Add the mixed vegetables and stir-fry for 3-4 minutes, or until tender.
3) Add the cooked brown rice and tamari sauce to the skillet and stir to combine.
4) Cook for an additional 1-2 minutes, or until everything is heated through.
5) Season with salt and pepper to taste.

Chapter 2: Lunch and Dinner Ideas

SOUPS AND STEWS

Carrot and Ginger Soup

Ingredients:

- 4 cups of chopped carrots
- 1 tablespoon of grated fresh ginger
- 1 tablespoon of olive oil
- 3 cups of low-sodium chicken or vegetable broth
- Salt and pepper to taste

Cooking Guidelines :

1) In a large pot, heat the olive oil over medium heat.

2) Add the chopped carrots and grated ginger and sauté for 5 minutes.
3) Add the chicken or vegetable broth and bring to a boil.
4) Reduce the heat to low and simmer for 15-20 minutes, or until the carrots are tender.
5) Use an immersion blender to puree the soup until smooth.
6) Season with salt and pepper to taste.

Chicken and Rice Soup

Ingredients:

- 1 pound of boneless, skinless chicken breast, cut into bite-sized pieces
- 1 cup of cooked white rice
- 3 cups of low-sodium chicken broth
- 1 cup of chopped carrots
- 1 cup of chopped celery
- 1 tablespoon of olive oil
- Salt and pepper to taste

Cooking Guidelines :

1) In a large pot, heat the olive oil over medium heat.
2) Add the chicken and sauté for 5-7 minutes, or until cooked through.
3) Add the chicken broth, chopped carrots, and chopped celery and bring to a boil.
4) Reduce the heat to low and simmer for 15-20 minutes, or until the vegetables are tender.
5) Stir in the cooked white rice and season with salt and pepper to taste.

Tomato and Basil Soup

Ingredients:

- 4 cups of canned crushed tomatoes
- 1/2 cup of chopped fresh basil
- 1 tablespoon of olive oil
- 3 cups of low-sodium chicken or vegetable broth
- Salt and pepper to taste

Cooking Guidelines :

1) In a large pot, heat the olive oil over medium heat.
2) Add the canned crushed tomatoes and chopped fresh basil and sauté for 5 minutes
3) Add the chicken or vegetable broth and bring to a boil.
4) Reduce the heat to low and simmer for 15-20 minutes, or until the soup has thickened slightly.
5) Season with salt and pepper to taste.

Lentil Stew

Ingredients:

- 2 cups of dried green lentils
- 1 cup of chopped carrots
- 1 cup of chopped celery
- 1 cup of chopped onion
- 3 cloves of garlic, minced
- 1 tablespoon of olive oil
- 4 cups of low-sodium chicken or vegetable broth
- Salt and pepper to taste

Cooking Guidelines :

1) In a large pot, heat the olive oil over medium heat.
2) Add the chopped onion and minced garlic and sauté for 2-3 minutes.
3) Add the chopped carrots and celery and sauté for 5 minutes.
4) Add the dried lentils and chicken or vegetable broth and bring to a boil.
5) Reduce the heat to low and simmer for 30-40 minutes, or until the lentils are tender.
6) Season with salt and pepper to taste.

Butternut Squash Soup

Ingredients:

- 4 cups of peeled and cubed butternut squash
- 1 tablespoon of grated fresh ginger
- 1 tablespoon of olive oil
- 3 cups of low-sodium chicken or vegetable broth
- Salt and pepper to taste

Cooking Guidelines :

1) In a large pot, heat the olive oil over medium heat.
2) Add the cubed butternut squash and grated fresh ginger and sauté for 5 minutes.
3) Add the chicken or vegetable broth and bring to a boil.
4) Reduce the heat to low and simmer for 20-25 minutes, or until the butternut squash is tender.
5) Use an immersion blender to puree the soup until smooth.
6) Season with salt and pepper to taste. Optional: garnish with a sprinkle of cinnamon or nutmeg before serving.

SLOW-COOKER MEALS

Slow-Cooker Chicken Tacos

Ingredients:

- 1 pound of boneless, skinless chicken breasts
- 1 onion, chopped
- 1 green bell pepper, chopped
- 1 red bell pepper, chopped
- 1 can of diced tomatoes
- 1 tablespoon of chili powder
- 1 teaspoon of ground cumin
- Salt and pepper to taste
- Corn tortillas, for serving
- Toppings such as diced avocado, shredded lettuce, and salsa (optional)

Cooking Guidelines :

1) Add the chicken breasts to the slow cooker and season with chili powder, ground cumin, salt, and pepper.
2) Add the chopped onion, green bell pepper, and red bell pepper to the slow cooker.
3) Pour the can of diced tomatoes over the top.
4) Cover and cook on low for 6-8 hours, or on high for 3-4 hours.
5) Once the chicken is cooked, use a fork to shred the meat in the slow cooker.
6) Serve the shredded chicken on corn tortillas with toppings of your choice.

Slow-Cooker Beef Stew

Ingredients:

- 1 pound of stew meat, cut into bite-sized pieces
- 1 onion, chopped
- 3 cloves of garlic, minced
- 2 cups of chopped carrots
- 2 cups of chopped potatoes
- 1 can of diced tomatoes
- 2 cups of low-sodium beef broth
- 1 tablespoon of Worcestershire sauce
- Salt and pepper to taste

Cooking Guidelines :

1) Add the stew meat to the slow cooker and season with salt and pepper.
2) Add the chopped onion, minced garlic, chopped carrots, and chopped potatoes to the slow cooker.
3) Pour the can of diced tomatoes and beef broth over the top.
4) Add Worcestershire sauce and stir to combine.
5) Cover and cook on low for 8-10 hours, or on high for 4-6 hours.
6) Serve hot.

Slow-Cooker Vegetable Soup

Ingredients:

- 4 cups of chopped mixed vegetables (such as carrots, celery, zucchini, and green beans)
- 1 onion, chopped

- 3 cloves of garlic, minced
- 1 can of diced tomatoes
- 4 cups of low-sodium vegetable broth
- 1 tablespoon of dried thyme
- Salt and pepper to taste

Cooking Guidelines :

1) Add the chopped mixed vegetables to the slow cooker.
2) Add the chopped onion and minced garlic to the slow cooker.
3) Pour the can of diced tomatoes and vegetable broth over the top.
4) Add dried thyme and stir to combine.
5) Cover and cook on low for 6-8 hours, or on high for 3-4 hours.
6) Serve hot.

Slow-Cooker Chili

Ingredients:

- 1 pound of ground beef or turkey
- 1 onion, chopped
- 3 cloves of garlic, minced
- 2 cans of kidney beans, drained and rinsed
- 1 can of diced tomatoes
- 1 can of tomato sauce
- 2 tablespoons of chili powder
- 1 teaspoon of ground cumin
- Salt and pepper to taste

Cooking Guidelines :

1) Brown the ground beef or turkey in a skillet over medium heat. Drain any excess fat.
2) Add the browned meat to the slow cooker.
3) Add the chopped onion and minced garlic to the slow cooker.
4) Pour the cans of kidney beans, diced tomatoes, and tomato sauce over the top.
5) Add chili powder and ground cumin and stir to combine.
6) Cover and cook on low for 6-8 hours, or on high for 3-4 hours.
7) Serve hot with toppings such as shredded cheese, diced avocado, and sour cream (optional).

Slow-Cooker Chicken and Rice Casserole

Ingredients:

- 1 pound of boneless, skinless chicken breasts
- 1 onion, chopped
- 1 green bell pepper, chopped
- 1 red bell pepper, chopped
- 1 can of diced tomatoes
- 2 cups of low-sodium chicken broth
- 1 cup of uncooked brown rice
- 1 tablespoon of dried oregano
- Salt and pepper to taste

Cooking Guidelines :

1) Add the chicken breasts to the slow cooker and season with dried oregano, salt, and pepper.
2) Add the chopped onion, green bell pepper, and red bell pepper to the slow cooker.

3) Pour the can of diced tomatoes and chicken broth over the top.
4) Add the uncooked brown rice and stir to combine.
5) Cover and cook on low for 6-8 hours, or on high for 3-4 hours.
6) Once the chicken and rice are cooked, use a fork to shred the chicken in the slow cooker.
7) Serve hot.

Chapter 3: Snacks and Appetizers

SMOOTHIES AND SHAKES

Apple Cinnamon Smoothie Basic

Ingredients:

- 1 cup unsweetened almond milk
- 1/2 cup unsweetened applesauce
- 1/2 banana
- 1 tsp cinnamon
- 1 tbsp maple syrup (optional)

Cooking Guidelines :

1) Combine all ingredients in a blender and blend until

smooth.

Apple Cinnamon Smoothie Bowl

Ingredients:

- 1 Apple Cinnamon Smoothie
- 1/4 cup gluten-free rolled oats
- 1 tbsp chia seeds
- 1 tbsp hemp seeds
- 1 tbsp unsweetened shredded coconut
- 1/4 cup fresh berries (such as blueberries or strawberries)
- 1 tbsp almond butter

Cooking Guidelines :

1) In a small bowl, combine the rolled oats, chia seeds, hemp seeds, and shredded coconut. Mix well.
2) Pour the Apple Cinnamon Smoothie into a bowl.
3) Top the smoothie with the oat mixture, fresh berries, and almond butter.

Apple Cinnamon Yogurt Dip

Ingredients:

- 1/2 cup plain Greek yogurt
- 1/2 cup unsweetened applesauce
- 1 tsp cinnamon
- 1/4 tsp nutmeg
- Apple slices or gluten-free crackers, for serving

Cooking Guidelines :

1) In a small bowl, mix together the Greek yogurt, applesauce, cinnamon, and nutmeg.
2) Serve the dip with apple slices or gluten-free crackers.

Avocado and Tomato Salad Basic

Ingredients:

- 1 ripe avocado, diced
- 1 ripe tomato, diced
- 1/4 red onion, thinly sliced
- 1 tbsp olive oil
- 1 tbsp fresh lime juice
- Salt and pepper to taste

Cooking Guidelines :

1) In a medium bowl, combine the diced avocado, diced tomato, and sliced red onion.
2) Drizzle with olive oil and lime juice and toss gently to combine.
3) Season with salt and pepper to taste.
4) Serve or chill until ready to serve.

Avocado and Tomato Salad with Shrimp

Ingredients:

- 1 Avocado and Tomato Salad
- 1/4 lb cooked shrimp, peeled and deveined
- 1 tbsp olive oil

- Salt and pepper to taste

Cooking Guidelines :

1) Prepare the Avocado and Tomato Salad according to the recipe below.
2) In a small pan, heat the olive oil over medium heat.
3) Add the cooked shrimp to the pan and season with salt and pepper to taste. Cook for 1-2 minutes until heated through.
4) Top the Avocado and Tomato Salad with the cooked shrimp.

Avocado and Tomato Salad Recipe

Ingredients:

- 1 ripe avocado, diced
- 1 ripe tomato, diced
- 1/4 red onion, thinly sliced
- 1 tbsp olive oil
- 1 tbsp fresh lime juice
- Salt and pepper to taste

Cooking Guidelines :

1) In a medium bowl, combine the diced avocado, diced tomato, and sliced red onion.
2) Drizzle with olive oil and lime juice and toss gently to combine.
3) Season with salt and pepper to taste.
4) Serve or chill until ready to serve.

Avocado and Tomato Salad Stuffed Cucumbers

Ingredients:

- 2 medium cucumbers, peeled and halved lengthwise
- 1 Avocado and Tomato Salad

Cooking Guidelines :

1) Scoop out the seeds and flesh from the center of each cucumber half, leaving a hollow cavity.
2) Fill each cucumber half with the Avocado and Tomato Salad.
3) Slice each cucumber half into 1-inch pieces.
4) Serve or chill until ready to serve.

Greek Yogurt and Berry Parfait

Ingredients:

- 1/2 cup plain Greek yogurt
- 1/4 cup gluten-free granola
- 1/2 cup mixed fresh berries (such as blueberries, raspberries, and strawberries)
- 1 tbsp honey (optional)

Cooking Guidelines :

1) In a small bowl, layer the Greek yogurt, granola, and mixed berries.
2) Drizzle with honey, if desired.
3) Serve or chill until ready to serve.

Greek Yogurt and Berry Dip

Ingredients:

- 1/2 cup plain Greek yogurt
- 1/4 cup mixed fresh berries (such as blueberries, raspberries, and strawberries), chopped
- 1 tbsp honey (optional)
- Gluten-free crackers or apple slices, for serving

Cooking Guidelines :

1) In a small bowl, mix together the Greek yogurt, chopped mixed berries, and honey.
2) Serve the dip with gluten-free crackers or apple slices.

Hummus Basic

Ingredients:

- 1 can (15 oz) chickpeas, drained and rinsed
- 2 cloves garlic, minced
- 2 tbsp tahini
- 2 tbsp olive oil
- 1 tbsp fresh lemon juice
- 1/2 tsp ground cumin
- Salt and pepper to taste

Cooking Guidelines :

1) In a food processor, combine the chickpeas, garlic, tahini, olive oil, lemon juice, and cumin.
2) Process until smooth, scraping down the sides of the bowl as needed
3) Season with salt and pepper to taste.

4) If the hummus is too thick, add water 1 tablespoon at a time until the desired consistency is reached.

Carrot and Hummus Stuffed Cucumber Cups

Ingredients:

- 2 medium cucumbers
- 1/2 cup hummus (store-bought or homemade)
- 1 large carrot, shredded
- 1 tbsp chopped fresh parsley

Cooking Guidelines :

1) Peel the cucumbers and cut them into 1-inch pieces.
2) Using a small spoon or melon baller, scoop out the center of each cucumber piece to create a hollow cup.
3) Fill each cucumber cup with a spoonful of hummus.
4) Top the hummus with a sprinkle of shredded carrot and chopped fresh parsley.
5) Serve or chill until ready to serve.

Carrot Sticks with Hummus Dip

Ingredients:

- 4 large carrots, peeled and cut into sticks
- 1/2 cup hummus (store-bought or homemade)

Cooking Guidelines :

1) Arrange the carrot sticks on a plate or platter.
2) Serve the hummus on the side for dipping.

Cucumber and Tuna Salad Bites

Ingredients:

- 1 can (5 oz) tuna, drained and flaked
- 2 tbsp mayonnaise (or Greek yogurt for a lighter option)
- 1 tsp Dijon mustard
- 1/2 small red onion, finely chopped
- 1 small celery stalk, finely chopped
- 1 small carrot, finely chopped
- Salt and pepper to taste
- 2 medium cucumbers, sliced into rounds
- Fresh parsley, for garnish

Cooking Guidelines :

1) In a medium bowl, mix together the tuna, mayonnaise, Dijon mustard, red onion, celery, and carrot.
2) Season with salt and pepper to taste.
3) Arrange the cucumber rounds on a platter.
4) Spoon a small amount of the tuna salad onto each cucumber round.
5) Garnish with fresh parsley.
6) Serve or chill until ready to serve.

NUTRITIOUS DIPS AND SPREADS

Roasted Red Pepper Hummus

Ingredients:

- 1 can (15 oz) chickpeas, drained and rinsed
- 1/2 cup roasted red peppers, drained
- 2 cloves garlic, minced
- 2 tbsp tahini
- 2 tbsp olive oil
- 1 tbsp fresh lemon juice
- 1/2 tsp ground cumin
- Salt and pepper to taste

Cooking Guidelines :

1) In a food processor, combine the chickpeas, roasted red peppers, garlic, tahini, olive oil, lemon juice, and cumin.
2) Process until smooth, scraping down the sides of the bowl as needed.
3) Season with salt and pepper to taste.
4) If the hummus is too thick, add water 1 tablespoon at a time until the desired consistency is reached.
5) Transfer the hummus to a serving bowl.
6) Garnish with additional roasted red peppers and a drizzle of olive oil, if desired.
7) Serve with gluten-free crackers or vegetable sticks for dipping.

Avocado and Tomato Salsa

Ingredients:

- 1 large avocado, diced
- 2 medium tomatoes, diced
- 1/2 small red onion, finely chopped
- 1 small jalapeño pepper, seeded and finely chopped

- 2 tbsp chopped fresh cilantro
- 1 tbsp fresh lime juice
- Salt and pepper to taste

Cooking Guidelines :

1) In a medium bowl, combine the diced avocado, diced tomatoes, red onion, jalapeño pepper, and chopped cilantro.
2) Drizzle with fresh lime juice and season with salt and pepper to taste.
3) Gently stir the ingredients together until well combined.
4) Serve or chill until ready to serve.
5) Eat with gluten-free crackers, tortilla chips, or as a topping for grilled fish or chicken.

Olive Tapenade

Ingredients:

- 1 cup pitted Kalamata olives
- 1/4 cup chopped fresh parsley
- 2 tbsp capers
- 2 cloves garlic, minced
- 2 tbsp fresh lemon juice
- 2 tbsp olive oil
- Salt and pepper to taste

Cooking Guidelines :

1) In a food processor, combine the Kalamata olives, chopped parsley, capers, minced garlic, fresh lemon juice, and olive oil.

2) Process until the mixture is smooth, scraping down the sides of the bowl as needed.
3) Season with salt and pepper to taste.
4) Transfer the olive tapenade to a serving bowl.
5) Garnish with additional chopped parsley and a drizzle of olive oil, if desired.
6) Serve with gluten-free crackers, cucumber slices, or as a topping for grilled chicken or fish.

White Bean Dip

Ingredients:

- 1 can (15 oz) cannellini beans, drained and rinsed
- 1/4 cup fresh parsley leaves
- 2 tbsp fresh lemon juice
- 2 cloves garlic, minced
- 1/4 tsp smoked paprika
- 2 tbsp olive oil
- Salt and pepper to taste

Cooking Guidelines :

1) In a food processor, combine the cannellini beans, fresh parsley leaves, fresh lemon juice, minced garlic, smoked paprika, and olive oil.
2) Process until the mixture is smooth, scraping down the sides of the bowl as needed.
3) Season with salt and pepper to taste.
4) If the dip is too thick, add water 1 tablespoon at a time until the desired consistency is reached.
5) Transfer the white bean dip to a serving bowl.
6) Garnish with additional parsley leaves and a drizzle of olive oil, if desired.

7) Serve with gluten-free crackers or vegetable sticks for dipping.

Cashew Cheese Dip

Ingredients:

- 1 cup raw cashews, soaked in water for at least 2 hours
- 2 tbsp nutritional yeast
- 1 clove garlic, minced
- 1/4 cup water
- 2 tbsp fresh lemon juice
- 1/4 tsp salt

Cooking Guidelines :

1) Drain and rinse the soaked cashews.
2) In a food processor, combine the cashews, nutritional yeast, minced garlic, water, fresh lemon juice, and salt.
3) Process until the mixture is smooth and creamy, scraping down the sides of the bowl as needed.
4) If the dip is too thick, add water 1 tablespoon at a time until the desired consistency is reached.
5) Transfer the cashew cheese dip to a serving bowl.
6) Garnish with chopped fresh herbs, if desired.
7) Serve with gluten-free crackers, sliced vegetables, or as a spread for sandwiches.

BAKED FOODS

Gluten-Free Banana Muffins

Ingredients:

- 2 cups gluten-free all-purpose flour
- 1/2 cup coconut sugar
- 1 tsp baking powder
- 1 tsp baking soda
- 1/2 tsp salt
- 1/2 cup unsweetened applesauce
- 2 ripe bananas, mashed
- 1/4 cup coconut oil, melted
- 1 tsp vanilla extract
- 2 large eggs, lightly beaten

Cooking Guidelines :

1) Preheat the oven to 350°F (180°C). Line a muffin tin with paper liners or grease with cooking spray.
2) In a large mixing bowl, combine the gluten-free all-purpose flour, coconut sugar, baking powder, baking soda, and salt.
3) In a separate mixing bowl, combine the unsweetened applesauce, mashed bananas, melted coconut oil, vanilla extract, and lightly beaten eggs.
4) Pour the wet ingredients into the dry ingredients and stir until just combined.
5) Divide the batter evenly between the muffin cups, filling each about 3/4 full.
6) Bake for 20-25 minutes, or until a toothpick inserted into the center of a muffin comes out clean.
7) Allow the muffins to cool in the tin for 5 minutes, then transfer to a wire rack to cool completely.

Almond Flour Crackers

Ingredients:

- 1 1/2 cups almond flour
- 1/2 tsp baking soda
- 1/4 tsp salt
- 1/4 tsp garlic powder
- 1/4 tsp onion powder
- 2 tbsp olive oil
- 2 tbsp water

Cooking Guidelines :

1) Preheat the oven to 350°F (180°C). Line a baking sheet with parchment paper.
2) In a mixing bowl, combine the almond flour, baking soda, salt, garlic powder, and onion powder.
3) Add the olive oil and water to the dry ingredients and mix until a dough forms.
4) Place the dough on a sheet of parchment paper and place another sheet on top.
5) Use a rolling pin to roll out the dough to about 1/8-inch thickness.
6) Use a knife or pizza cutter to cut the dough into small squares or rectangles.
7) Transfer the crackers to the prepared baking sheet, leaving a little space between each cracker.
8) Bake for 12-15 minutes, or until the crackers are golden brown and crispy.
9) Allow the crackers to cool on the baking sheet for 5 minutes, then transfer to a wire rack to cool completely.
10) Serve the almond flour crackers with your favorite dips, spreads, or cheeses.

Quinoa and Vegetable Mini Frittatas

Ingredients:

- 1/2 cup quinoa, cooked
- 1/2 cup zucchini, grated
- 1/2 cup red bell pepper, diced
- 1/4 cup scallions, chopped
- 1/4 cup fresh parsley, chopped
- 1/2 tsp salt
- 1/4 tsp black pepper
- 4 large eggs, beaten

Cooking Guidelines :

1) Preheat the oven to 375°F (190°C). Grease a mini muffin tin with cooking spray.
2) In a mixing bowl, combine the cooked quinoa, grated zucchini, diced red bell pepper, chopped scallions, and chopped parsley.
3) Add the salt and black pepper to the bowl and stir to combine.
4) Add the beaten eggs to the bowl and mix until everything is well combined.
5) Use a spoon to divide the mixture evenly among the muffin cups.
6) Bake for 15-20 minutes, or until the frittatas are set and lightly golden brown.
7) Allow the frittatas to cool in the tin for a few minutes, then remove them from the tin and transfer to a wire rack to cool completely.

Gluten-Free Zucchini Bread

Ingredients:

- 1 1/2 cups gluten-free flour blend
- 1 tsp baking powder
- 1/2 tsp baking soda
- 1/2 tsp salt
- 1/2 tsp cinnamon
- 1/4 tsp nutmeg
- 1/4 cup coconut oil, melted
- 1/2 cup honey
- 2 large eggs
- 1 tsp vanilla extract
- 1 1/2 cups grated zucchini (about 1 medium zucchini)

Cooking Guidelines :

1) Preheat the oven to 350°F (180°C). Grease a 9x5 inch loaf pan with cooking spray.
2) In a mixing bowl, whisk together the gluten-free flour blend, baking powder, baking soda, salt, cinnamon, and nutmeg.
3) In another mixing bowl, beat together the melted coconut oil, honey, eggs, and vanilla extract.
4) Add the grated zucchini to the wet ingredients and stir to combine.
5) Gradually add the dry ingredients to the wet ingredients and stir until everything is well combined.
6) Pour the batter into the prepared loaf pan and spread it out evenly.
7) Bake for 45-50 minutes, or until a toothpick inserted into the center of the bread comes out clean.
8) Allow the bread to cool in the pan for 10-15 minutes, then remove it from the pan and transfer to a wire rack to cool completely.

9) Slice the gluten-free zucchini bread and serve it as a snack or for breakfast.

Carrot and Ginger Cookies

Ingredients:

- 1/2 cup almond flour
- 1/2 cup coconut flour
- 1 tsp baking powder
- 1/2 tsp baking soda
- 1/4 tsp salt
- 1 tsp ground cinnamon
- 1/2 tsp ground ginger
- 1/4 tsp ground nutmeg
- 1/4 cup coconut oil, melted
- 1/4 cup honey
- 1 large egg
- 1 tsp vanilla extract
- 1/2 cup grated carrots
- 1 tbsp grated fresh ginger

Cooking Guidelines :

1) Preheat the oven to 350°F (180°C). Line a baking sheet with parchment paper.
2) In a mixing bowl, whisk together the almond flour, coconut flour, baking powder, baking soda, salt, cinnamon, ginger, and nutmeg.
3) In another mixing bowl, beat together the melted coconut oil, honey, egg, and vanilla extract.
4) Add the grated carrots and fresh ginger to the wet ingredients and stir to combine.

5) Gradually add the dry ingredients to the wet ingredients and stir until everything is well combined.
6) Use a cookie scoop or spoon to drop balls of the dough onto the prepared baking sheet.
7) Use your fingers to flatten each ball into a cookie shape.
8) Bake for 12-15 minutes, or until the cookies are lightly golden brown.
9) Allow the cookies to cool on the baking sheet for a few minutes, then transfer them to a wire rack to cool completely.

PROTEIN BARS AND BITES

No-Bake Almond Butter Bars

Ingredients:

- 1 cup almond flour
- 1/2 cup almond butter
- 1/4 cup honey
- 1/4 cup coconut oil, melted
- 1 tsp vanilla extract
- 1/4 tsp salt
- 1/4 cup chopped almonds

Cooking Guidelines :

1) Line an 8x8 inch baking dish with parchment paper.
2) In a mixing bowl, stir together the almond flour, almond butter, honey, melted coconut oil, vanilla extract, and salt until well combined.
3) Fold in the chopped almonds.

4) Transfer the mixture to the prepared baking dish and use your fingers to press it down into an even layer.
5) Place the baking dish in the refrigerator and chill for at least 1 hour, or until the mixture is firm.
6) Use a sharp knife to cut the mixture into bars.

Blueberry Energy Bites

Ingredients:

- 1 cup gluten-free rolled oats
- 1/2 cup almond butter
- 1/4 cup honey
- 1/2 cup fresh blueberries, mashed
- 1/4 cup chopped almonds
- 1 tsp vanilla extract
- Pinch of salt

Cooking Guidelines :

1) In a mixing bowl, stir together the rolled oats, almond butter, honey, mashed blueberries, chopped almonds, vanilla extract, and salt until well combined.
2) Use a cookie scoop or spoon to portion the mixture into balls.
3) Use your hands to roll each portion into a ball.
4) Place the balls on a plate or baking sheet lined with parchment paper.
5) Chill the blueberry energy bites in the refrigerator for at least 30 minutes, or until they are firm.

Chocolate Peanut Butter Protein Bars

Ingredients:

- 1 cup gluten-free rolled oats
- 1/2 cup peanut butter
- 1/4 cup honey
- 1/4 cup unsweetened cocoa powder
- 1/4 cup vanilla protein powder
- 1/4 cup unsweetened almond milk
- 1/4 cup chopped peanuts
- Pinch of salt

Cooking Guidelines :

1) In a mixing bowl, stir together the rolled oats, peanut butter, honey, unsweetened cocoa powder, vanilla protein powder, almond milk, chopped peanuts, and salt until well combined.
2) Use a spatula to transfer the mixture to a 8x8 inch baking dish lined with parchment paper.
3) Use the spatula to spread the mixture out into an even layer.
4) Chill the mixture in the refrigerator for at least 1 hour, or until it is firm.
5) Use a sharp knife to cut the mixture into bars.

Cherry Vanilla Protein Bites

Ingredients:

- 1 cup gluten-free rolled oats
- 1/2 cup almond butter
- 1/4 cup honey
- 1/4 cup vanilla protein powder
- 1/4 cup chopped dried cherries

- 1 tsp vanilla extract
- Pinch of salt

Cooking Guidelines :

1) In a mixing bowl, stir together the rolled oats, almond butter, honey, vanilla protein powder, chopped dried cherries, vanilla extract, and salt until well combined.
2) Use a cookie scoop or spoon to portion the mixture into balls.
3) Use your hands to roll each portion into a ball.
4) Place the balls on a plate or baking sheet lined with parchment paper.
5) Chill the cherry vanilla protein bites in the refrigerator for at least 30 minutes, or until they are firm.

No-Bake Pumpkin Spice Bars

Ingredients:

- 1 1/2 cups gluten-free rolled oats
- 1/2 cup almond butter
- 1/4 cup honey
- 1/2 cup pumpkin puree
- 1/4 cup chopped pecans
- 1 tsp pumpkin pie spice
- Pinch of salt

Cooking Guidelines :

1) In a mixing bowl, stir together the rolled oats, almond butter, honey, pumpkin puree, chopped pecans, pumpkin pie spice, and salt until well combined.
2) Use a spatula to transfer the mixture to a 8x8 inch

baking dish lined with parchment paper.

3) Use the spatula to spread the mixture out into an even layer.

4) Chill the mixture in the refrigerator for at least 1 hour, or until it is firm.

5) Use a sharp knife to cut the mixture into bars.

Chapter 4: Beverages

SMOOTHIES AND SHAKES

Strawberry Banana Smoothie

Ingredients:

- 1 ripe banana
- 1 cup frozen strawberries
- 1/2 cup unsweetened almond milk
- 1/2 cup Greek yogurt
- 1 tsp honey (optional)
- 1/4 tsp vanilla extract
- Ice (optional)

Cooking Guidelines :

1) Add the ripe banana, frozen strawberries,

unsweetened almond milk, Greek yogurt, honey (if using), and vanilla extract to a blender.
2) Blend the ingredients until smooth.
3) If desired, add a handful of ice to the blender and blend until the smoothie reaches your desired consistency.
4) Pour the strawberry banana smoothie into a glass and serve immediately.
5) You can also add other ingredients like chia seeds, flaxseeds or spinach to make it more nutritious.

Blueberry Almond Milk Shake

Ingredients:

- 1 cup frozen blueberries
- 1/2 cup unsweetened almond milk
- 1/2 cup Greek yogurt
- 1 tsp honey (optional)
- 1/4 tsp vanilla extract
- Ice (optional)

Cooking Guidelines :

1) Add the frozen blueberries, unsweetened almond milk, Greek yogurt, honey (if using), and vanilla extract to a blender.
2) Blend the ingredients until smooth.
3) If desired, add a handful of ice to the blender and blend until the shake reaches your desired consistency.
4) Pour the blueberry almond milk shake into a glass and serve immediately.
5) You can also add other ingredients like chia seeds,

flaxseeds, or spinach to make it more nutritious.

Note: if you have trouble tolerating blueberries, you can substitute with another frozen fruit such as strawberries or raspberries.

Mango Lassi Smoothie

Ingredients:

- 1 ripe mango, peeled and diced
- 1/2 cup plain Greek yogurt
- 1/2 cup unsweetened almond milk
- 1 tsp honey (optional)
- 1/4 tsp ground cardamom
- Ice (optional)

Cooking Guidelines :

1) Add the diced mango, Greek yogurt, unsweetened almond milk, honey (if using), and ground cardamom to a blender.
2) Blend the ingredients until smooth.
3) If desired, add a handful of ice to the blender and blend until the smoothie reaches your desired consistency.
4) Pour the mango lassi smoothie into a glass and serve immediately.
5) You can also add other ingredients like chia seeds, flaxseeds, or spinach to make it more nutritious.

Note: if can't tolerating mango, you can substitute with another frozen fruit such as peaches or pineapple.

Chocolate Avocado Smoothie

Ingredients:

- 1/2 ripe avocado, pitted and peeled
- 1 cup unsweetened almond milk
- 1/2 cup plain Greek yogurt
- 1 tbsp unsweetened cocoa powder
- 1 tsp honey (optional)
- Ice (optional)

Cooking Guidelines :

1) Add the ripe avocado, unsweetened almond milk, plain Greek yogurt, unsweetened cocoa powder, and honey (if using) to a blender.
2) Blend the ingredients until smooth.
3) If desired, add a handful of ice to the blender and blend until the smoothie reaches your desired consistency.
4) Pour the chocolate avocado smoothie into a glass and serve immediately.
5) You can also add other ingredients like chia seeds, flaxseeds, or spinach to make it more nutritious.

Note: If you can't tolerating cocoa powder, you can substitute with carob powder which is a caffeine-free alternative.

Green Smoothie

Ingredients:

- 1 ripe banana
- 1/2 ripe avocado, pitted and peeled
- 1 cup baby spinach leaves

- 1/2 cup unsweetened almond milk
- 1/2 cup plain Greek yogurt
- 1 tsp honey (optional)
- Ice (optional)

Cooking Guidelines :

1) Add the ripe banana, ripe avocado, baby spinach leaves, unsweetened almond milk, plain Greek yogurt, and honey (if using) to a blender.
2) Blend the ingredients until smooth.
3) If desired, add a handful of ice to the blender and blend until the smoothie reaches your desired consistency.
4) Pour the green smoothie into a glass and serve immediately.
5) You can also add other ingredients like chia seeds, flaxseeds, or protein powder to make it more nutritious.

Note: if you can't tolerating spinach, you can substitute with kale or another leafy green vegetable.

JUICES AND HERBAL TEAS

Ginger Lemon Tea

Ingredients:

- 2-inch piece fresh ginger, peeled and sliced
- 1/2 lemon, juiced
- 2 cups water
- Honey (optional)

Cooking Guidelines :

1) Add the sliced fresh ginger and water to a small saucepan and bring to a boil.
2) Reduce heat and let the ginger simmer in the water for 10-15 minutes.
3) Remove the saucepan from heat and strain the ginger pieces from the water.
4) Stir in the fresh lemon juice and honey (if using) to taste.
5) Serve the ginger lemon tea hot in a mug.

Mint Green Tea

Ingredients:

- 2 green tea bags
- 4 cups water
- 1/4 cup fresh mint leaves
- Honey (optional)

Cooking Guidelines :

1) Add the water to a small saucepan and bring to a boil.
2) Remove from heat and add the green tea bags and fresh mint leaves to the hot water.
3) Let the tea steep for 3-5 minutes, or until it reaches the desired strength.
4) Remove the tea bags and strain the mint leaves from the tea.
5) Stir in honey (if using) to taste.
6) Serve the mint green tea hot in a mug.

Carrot Ginger Juice

Ingredients:

- 4 medium-sized carrots, peeled and chopped
- 1-inch piece fresh ginger, peeled and chopped
- 1/2 cup water
- Ice (optional)

Cooking Guidelines :

1) Add the chopped carrots, ginger, and water to a juicer and juice until the mixture is smooth.
2) If desired, add a handful of ice to the juice and blend until the juice reaches your desired consistency.
3) Pour the carrot ginger juice into a glass and serve immediately.
4) You can also add other ingredients like apples or oranges to make it more flavorful.

Note: If you don't have a juicer, you can use a blender instead. Simply blend the ingredients until smooth and strain the mixture through a fine-mesh sieve or cheesecloth to remove the pulp.

Apple Cider Vinegar Drink

Ingredients:

- 1-2 tablespoons of apple cider vinegar
- 8-10 ounces of water
- Honey or Stevia (optional)
- Dash of cinnamon (optional)

Cooking Guidelines :

1) Fill a glass with 8-10 ounces of water.
2) Add 1-2 tablespoons of apple cider vinegar to the water.
3) If desired, add honey or stevia to taste, and a dash of cinnamon for flavor.
4) Stir the mixture until the ingredients are well combined.
5) Serve the apple cider vinegar drink chilled or at room temperature.

Fennel Tea

Ingredients:

- 1-2 teaspoons fennel seeds
- 8-10 ounces of water
- Honey or Stevia (optional)

Cooking Guidelines :

1) Add 1-2 teaspoons of fennel seeds to a teapot or infuser.
2) Bring 8-10 ounces of water to a boil and pour the hot water over the fennel seeds.
3) Let the tea steep for 5-10 minutes, or until it reaches the desired strength.
4) Strain the tea through a fine-mesh sieve or cheesecloth to remove the fennel seeds.
5) If desired, add honey or stevia to taste.
6) Serve the fennel tea hot in a mug.

ELECTROLYTE DRINKS

Homemade Electrolyte Drink

Ingredients:

- 2 cups of filtered water
- 1/4 teaspoon of sea salt
- 1/4 teaspoon of baking soda
- 2 tablespoons of honey or maple syrup
- 1/2 cup of freshly squeezed orange juice
- 1/4 cup of freshly squeezed lemon juice

Cooking Guidelines :

1) Add 2 cups of filtered water to a pitcher.
2) Stir in 1/4 teaspoon of sea salt and 1/4 teaspoon of baking soda until they are fully dissolved.
3) Add 2 tablespoons of honey or maple syrup to the mixture and stir until dissolved.
4) Stir in 1/2 cup of freshly squeezed orange juice and 1/4 cup of freshly squeezed lemon juice.
5) Stir the mixture until all ingredients are fully combined.
6) Chill the mixture in the refrigerator for at least 30 minutes before serving.
7) Serve the electrolyte drink chilled or over ice.

Coconut Water and Pineapple Smoothie

Ingredients:

- 1 cup of coconut water
- 1 cup of fresh or frozen pineapple chunks
- 1/2 banana
- 1/2 cup of plain Greek yogurt

- 1/2 teaspoon of grated ginger (optional)
- 1/4 teaspoon of vanilla extract (optional)

Cooking Guidelines :

1) Add 1 cup of coconut water to a blender.
2) Add 1 cup of fresh or frozen pineapple chunks to the blender.
3) Slice 1/2 banana and add it to the blender.
4) Add 1/2 cup of plain Greek yogurt to the blender.
5) Add 1/2 teaspoon of grated ginger (optional) and 1/4 teaspoon of vanilla extract (optional) to the blender.
6) Blend all ingredients until smooth and creamy.
7) Taste the smoothie and adjust sweetness or consistency to your liking by adding honey, ice, or more fruit.
8) Serve the smoothie in a glass or to-go cup.

Berry Electrolyte Smoothie

Ingredients:

- 1 cup of coconut water
- 1 cup of frozen mixed berries (strawberries, raspberries, and blueberries)
- 1/2 banana
- 1/2 cup of plain Greek yogurt
- 1/4 teaspoon of vanilla extract (optional)
- 1 tablespoon of honey (optional)

Cooking Guidelines :

1) Add 1 cup of coconut water to a blender.
2) Add 1 cup of frozen mixed berries to the blender.

3) Slice 1/2 banana and add it to the blender.
4) Add 1/2 cup of plain Greek yogurt to the blender.
5) Add 1/4 teaspoon of vanilla extract (optional) and 1 tablespoon of honey (optional) to the blender.
6) Blend all ingredients until smooth and creamy.
7) Taste the smoothie and adjust sweetness or consistency to your liking by adding more honey or ice.
8) Serve the smoothie in a glass or to-go cup.

Lemon Lime Electrolyte Drink

Ingredients:

- 1 cup of coconut water
- Juice from 1 lemon
- Juice from 1 lime
- 1-2 tablespoons of honey (optional)
- Pinch of sea salt

Cooking Guidelines :

1) In a large glass, add 1 cup of coconut water.
2) Squeeze the juice from 1 lemon and 1 lime into the glass with the coconut water.
3) Add 1-2 tablespoons of honey (optional) to the glass and stir well.
4) Add a pinch of sea salt to the glass and stir well again.
5) Taste the drink and adjust sweetness or saltiness to your liking.
6) Serve the drink over ice, if desired.

Chia Seed Electrolyte Drink

Ingredients:

- 1 tablespoon of chia seeds
- 1 cup of coconut water
- Juice from 1 lemon
- 1-2 teaspoons of honey (optional)
- Pinch of sea salt

Cooking Guidelines :

1) In a small bowl, add 1 tablespoon of chia seeds and 1/4 cup of water. Stir well and let the mixture sit for 10-15 minutes, or until the chia seeds have absorbed the water and formed a gel-like texture.
2) In a large glass, add 1 cup of coconut water.
3) Squeeze the juice from 1 lemon into the glass with the coconut water.
4) Add 1-2 teaspoons of honey (optional) to the glass and stir well.
5) Add a pinch of sea salt to the glass and stir well again.
6) Once the chia seed mixture has formed a gel-like texture, add it to the glass with the electrolyte drink and stir well.
7) Taste the drink and adjust sweetness or saltiness to your liking.
8) Serve the drink over ice, if desired.

LOW-SUGAR COCKTAILS

Vodka Soda with Lime

Ingredients:

- 1.5 oz of vodka
- Soda water
- Juice from 1 lime
- Ice

Cooking Guidelines :

1) Fill a glass with ice.
2) Add 1.5 oz of vodka to the glass.
3) Squeeze the juice from 1 lime into the glass.
4) Fill the glass with soda water.
5) Stir well.
6) Garnish with a lime wedge, if desired.

Tequila Sunrise

Ingredients:

- 1.5 oz of tequila
- 3 oz of fresh orange juice
- 1 oz of pomegranate juice
- Ice

Cooking Guidelines :

1) Fill a glass with ice.
2) Add 1.5 oz of tequila to the glass.
3) Pour in 3 oz of fresh orange juice.
4) Slowly pour in 1 oz of pomegranate juice to create the sunrise effect.
5) Stir gently.
6) Garnish with an orange slice, if desired.

Gin and Tonic with Cucumber

Ingredients:

- 1.5 oz of gin
- Tonic water
- Sliced cucumber
- Ice

Cooking Guidelines :

1) Fill a glass with ice.
2) Add 1.5 oz of gin to the glass.
3) Fill the glass with tonic water.
4) Stir gently.
5) Add a few slices of cucumber to the glass.
6) Stir again.

Skinny Margarita

Ingredients:

- 1.5 oz of silver tequila
- 1 oz of fresh lime juice
- 1/2 oz of agave nectar
- Salt for rim (optional)
- Ice

Cooking Guidelines :

1) Rim a glass with salt (optional).
2) Fill the glass with ice.
3) In a shaker, combine 1.5 oz of silver tequila, 1 oz of fresh lime juice, and 1/2 oz of agave nectar.
4) Shake well.

5) Pour the mixture over the ice in the glass.

Strawberry Basil Smash

Ingredients:

- 4-5 strawberries, hulled and chopped
- 3-4 basil leaves
- 1 oz of fresh lemon juice
- 1/2 oz of agave nectar
- 1.5 oz of gin
- Soda water
- Ice

Cooking Guidelines :

1) In a shaker, muddle 4-5 strawberries and 3-4 basil leaves.
2) Add 1 oz of fresh lemon juice and 1/2 oz of agave nectar to the shaker.
3) Add 1.5 oz of gin and shake well.
4) Fill a glass with ice and strain the mixture from the shaker into the glass.
5) Top with soda water and stir.
6) Garnish with a strawberry or basil leaf (optional).

ABOUT THE AUTHOR

Aashvi Dhingra is an India born woman who currently resides in the United States. Aashvi has always been passionate about food and nutrition, which led her to pursue a career as a Registered Dietitian. Aashvi earned her Bachelor's degree in Nutrition and Dietetics from a prestigious university in India, and later received her Master's degree in Nutrition Science from a renowned university in the United States.

Aashvi's journey as a dietitian began in India, where she worked in various clinical and community settings. During her time in India, Aashvi developed a keen interest in the intersection between food, culture, and health. She conducted several research studies on the impact of traditional Indian diets on health outcomes, which earned her recognition and awards from various academic and research organizations.

In the United States, Aashvi has worked as a clinical dietitian in a hospital setting, where she has helped patients with various health conditions achieve their nutrition goals. Aashvi has also worked with several community organizations to promote healthy eating habits and improve access to nutritious foods.

Apart from her professional work as a dietitian, Aashvi is an avid home cook who loves experimenting with new recipes and flavors. She believes that cooking is a creative and therapeutic process that brings people together and fosters cultural exchange. Aashvi often shares her recipes and cooking tips on her social media platforms and has gained a significant following.

Aashvi's multicultural background and experience as a dietitian have shaped her approach to food and nutrition. She believes that a healthy and balanced diet should be personalized to an individual's cultural background, preferences, and lifestyle. Aashvi also emphasizes the importance of food education and empowering individuals to make informed choices about their diet.

Through her work as a dietitian and her passion for cooking, Aashvi hopes to inspire others to prioritize their health and well-being through food. She also aims to promote cultural understanding and celebrate the diversity of cuisines and culinary traditions around the world.

In her free time, Aashvi enjoys traveling, hiking, and exploring new restaurants and food markets. She is also an avid reader and enjoys learning about new topics related to food, culture, and health.